Sugar Detox Guide

Beat Cravings and Lose Weight in 21 Days Or Less

Busting Sugar Addiction with 30 Great Sugar Detox Recipes and Diet Plans

By: Ethan Owen

PUBLISHERS NOTES

This book is copyright © 2014 by ETHAN OWEN.

This publication is intended to provide helpful and informative material. It is not intended to diagnose, treat, cure, or prevent any health problem or condition, nor is intended to replace the advice of a physician. No action should be taken solely on the contents of this book. Always consult your physician or qualified health-care professional on any matters regarding your health and before adopting any suggestions in this book or drawing inferences from it.

The author and publisher specifically disclaim all responsibility for any liability, loss or risk, personal or otherwise, which is incurred as a consequence, directly or indirectly, from the use or application of any contents of this book.

Any and all product names referenced within this book are the trademark of their respective owners. None of these owners have sponsored, authorized, endorsed, or approved this book.

Always read all information provided by the manufacturers' product labels before using their products. The author and publisher are not responsible for claims made by manufacturers.

Published by:
SPEEDY PUBLISHING LLC
40 E MAIN ST, #1156
NEWARK, DELAWARE 19711
Paperback Edition

Manufactured in the United States of America

What You Will Learn In This Book

How This Book Will Help You and Why

This book will provide you with a practical and sound way of getting over sugar addiction. You can learn simple and straightforward ways of being able to beat those pesky sugar cravings. By following what you will learn in this book you can wean yourself of sweet foods and protect yourself from things such as diabetes and heart disease.

TABLE OF CONTENTS

Publishers Notes	2
What You Will Learn In This Book	3
Dedication	7
1 Let's Start By Detoxing	8
2 Reenergize and Revitalize with Vitamins	14
3 Start Eating More Fruit : The Best Start to Your New Diet	20
4 Boosting Your Diet with Superfoods : Forget That Sugar!	26
5 Do Not Hold The Horses!	32
6 Coffee, Coffee and Coffee!	37
7 The Secret Foods That Busts Sugar	44
8 Get Rid Of The Msg : This Is The Final Tip For Sugar Busting	49
The Most Important Thing You Can Do To Spread The Word	55
About The Author	57

DEDICATION

This book is dedicated to anyone that has struggled with any addiction in their lives. There is hope for you yet and will power to overcome is the best cure for any disease.

> *Success is to be measured not so much by the position that one has reached in life as by the obstacles which he has overcome.*

- **Booker T. Washington**

1 LET'S START BY DETOXING

. . .

To begin the process of the sugar detox you must first start with antioxidants. If you don't it renders the whole process useless. You must first start to bring you blood sugar levels back inline. Let's look on a bit more about antioxidants.

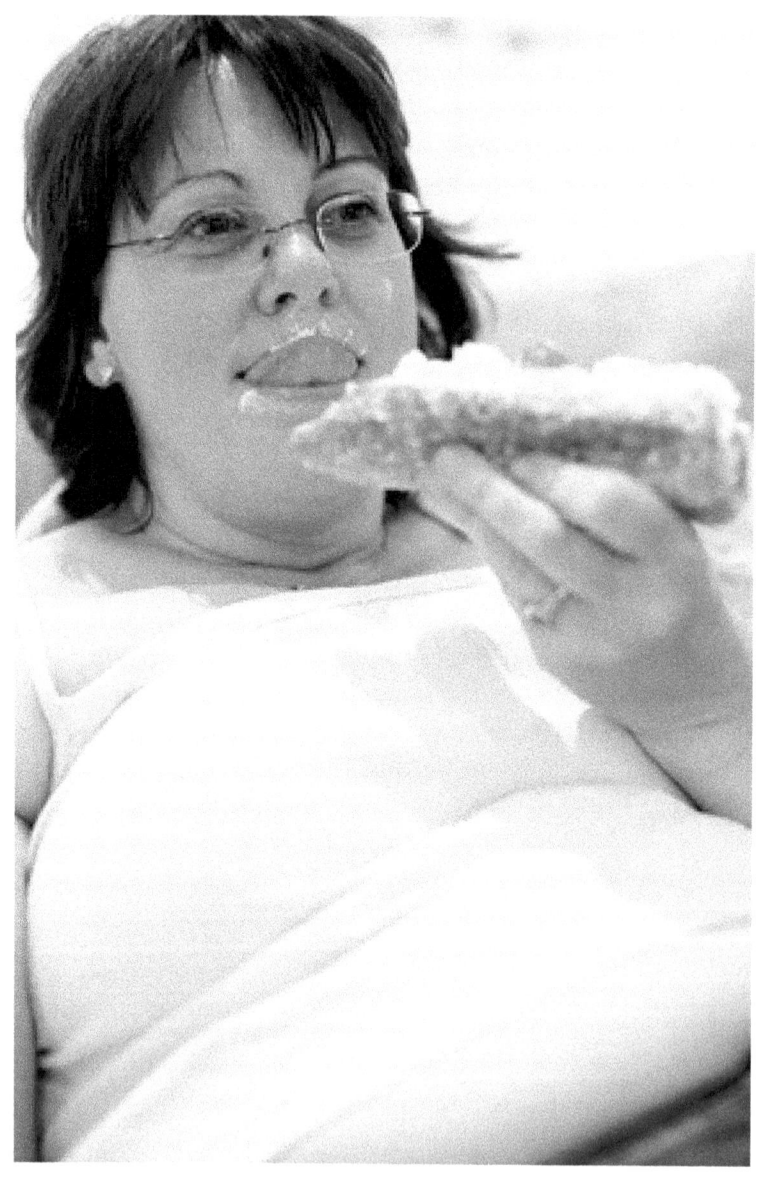

Most people know that antioxidants neutralize the free radicals that damage cells and contribute to diseases like cancers, heart disease, arthritis, and many other conditions. Antioxidants contribute to a feeling of vitality and health, and they ward off the effects of aging.

There are plenty of antioxidant supplements available, but nutritionists and health experts agree that obtaining antioxidants from food is the best approach. This need not be a chore or dull, because antioxidants are found in all kinds of foods, and even in coffee and black chocolate! I don't know about you, but you won't have to twist my arm to have a piece of dark chocolate every day!

One of the best sources of antioxidants is colorful fruits and vegetables. As a rule, the more brightly colored, the higher the antioxidant content. If you choose fresh, colorful vegetables and fruits and make sure your diet has plenty of variety and few processed 'industrial' foods, you should have no trouble getting enough antioxidants.

The old saying that a plate of food should have something red, something green and something yellow or orange, is a sure way of selecting antioxidant-rich foods. Another old saying: "an apple a day keeps the doctor away" is also true, because apples (particularly the peel) contain huge amounts of antioxidants.

Berries of all kinds contain massive amounts of antioxidants called flavonoids. One thing to keep in mind, however, is that milk; cream, ice cream and other milk products interfere with antioxidants and prevent them working effectively, so serve your berries without the cream. (Sugar does not affect antioxidants.)

Cooked tomatoes contain a powerful antioxidant called lycopene. Vitamin content is often reduced through cooking foods, so generally raw fruits and vegetables, or those quickly stir-fried contain more antioxidants, but tomatoes are an exception.

Fresh, raw tomatoes do contain antioxidants in the form of vitamins, but products such as tomato paste, ketchup, tomato soup, and canned tomatoes contain more useful antioxidants because lycopene changes to a more useful form for the body when it is heated.

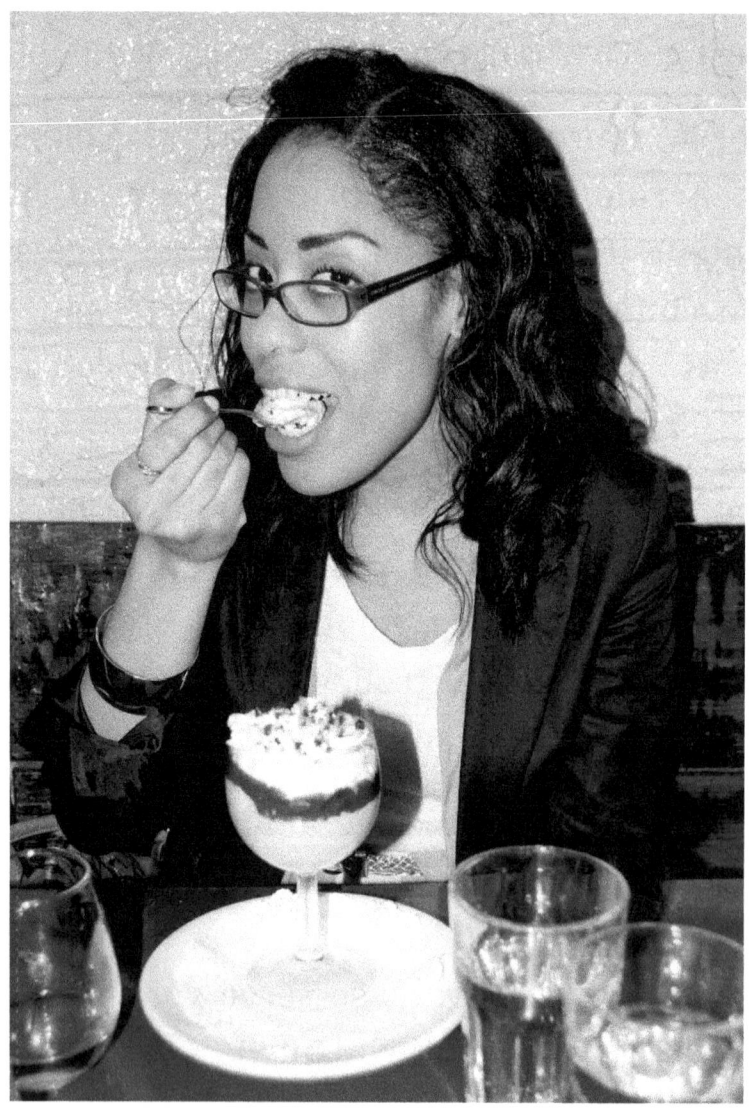

Team cooked tomatoes with garlic and onions to give you an antioxidant boost, because garlic and onions contain selenium, which forms part of powerful antioxidant proteins called selenoproteins. Fresh garlic and onions contain many other useful nutrients that have been shown to reduce cancers, lower blood pressure, and lower cholesterol levels, and garlic is also well known as a natural antibiotic.

Dried fruits and nuts are great sources of antioxidants. Brazil nuts are especially rich in selenium, which is a potent antioxidant, but all nuts and dried fruits contain good quantities of antioxidants. If you are thinking of a snack, fresh or dried fruits or nuts, are hard to beat.

Other good sources of antioxidants are tea, coffee and chocolate! Both green and black teas contain antioxidants, but if black tea is drunk with milk, the milk reduces the effectiveness of the antioxidants.

The same applies to coffee and chocolate, which also contain large quantities of antioxidants. So learn to like your tea, coffee and chocolate black. Incidentally, decaffeinated coffee also contains antioxidants.

Herbs such as parsley, sage, dill and oregano are also a good source of antioxidants, so remember to use them in your cooking and as garnishes. Most spices also contain antioxidants.

An unusual source of antioxidants is chia seeds (Salvia hispanica), which is sold in some health food stores. These tiny seeds are a good source of omega-3 fatty acids, which give added health benefits.

They contain soluble fiber, which lowers 'bad' LDL cholesterol levels in the blood, and early results of studies suggest they lower triglycerides and increase 'good' HDL cholesterol.

You can sprinkle chia seeds on breads, yoghurt, salads, or muffins, for example I will also put some in my soups and stews and have even mixed them will my home made jelly.

Another unusual source is krill, which are the tiny crustaceans some whales eat.

In many countries krill is seen only in fishing bait or aquarium fish food, but in Japan it is served in restaurants and is called okiami. Krill, or more specifically krill oil, contains astaxanthin, which is a very powerful antioxidant.

Lobster, shrimp and prawn also contain astaxanthin, which is the pigment that gives these crustaceans their red or pink color. Astanxanthin has the particularly useful property of being able to cross the blood-brain barrier, and this means it may be particularly effective in protecting against diseases such as Alzheimer's.

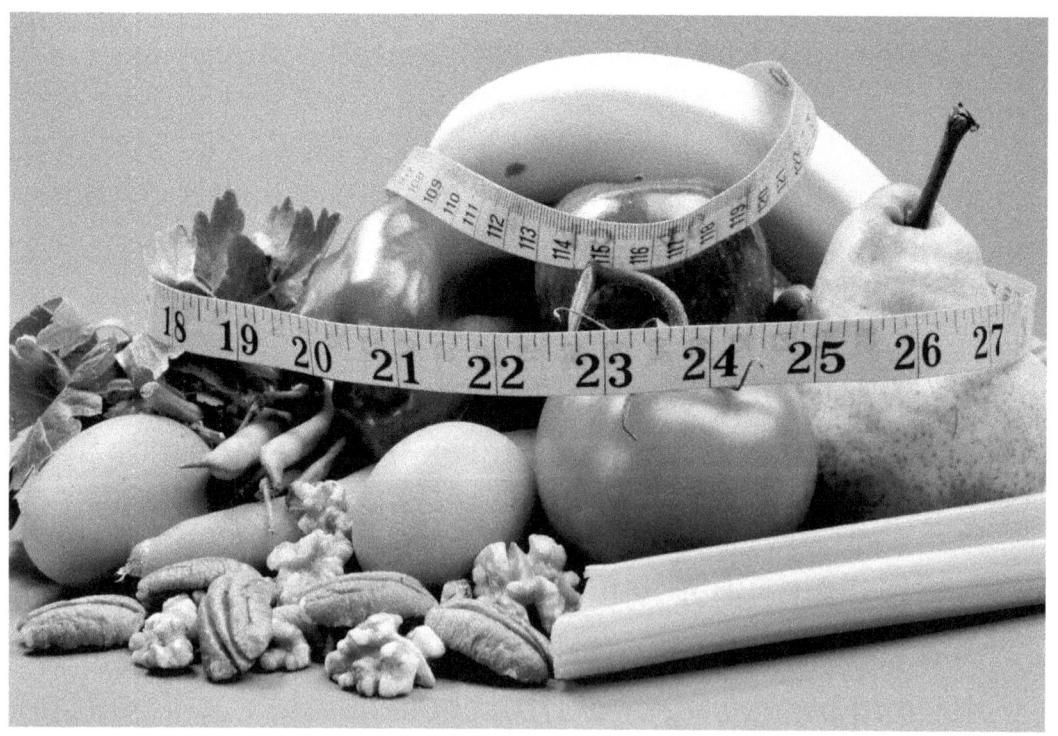

Antioxidants are vital nutrients in the fight against disease and the processes of aging. It is fortunate there are many natural, and often cheap sources of antioxidants and you do not have to make your meals dull. In fact doing the opposite and making meals colorful affairs full of variety and taste is guaranteed to boost your antioxidant intake. And don't forget the chocolate, but make it dark!

You may think the foods you can eat on your detox are boring or bland but try this, my favorite breakfast ever!

Butternut Squash with Green Apple and Smoked Ham Hash

Ingredients:
1 peeled/cubed medium Butternut Squash
1 or 2 Apples, I would go with the Granny Smith
A cup of smoked ham, cubed
Fresh green onions - a quarter cup chopped
1.5 teaspoons Italian seasoning

Sea salt and pepper as needed
2 or 3 tablespoons of oil, I like to use Coconut but any is fine

Get all the ingredients ready to go by chopping to the desired size.

Preheat your pan on a medium high setting. Add your oil to the bottom of the pan. Add in your squash, ham and the apples and fry all until golden.

Add the green onions and Italian seasoning along with salt and pepper to suit your taste and cook for another 5 minutes to allow everything to blend together.

Super easy and delicious!

Sugar Detox / Ethan Owen

2 REENERGIZE AND REVITALIZE WITH VITAMINS

. . .

One **major problem** with antioxidants and vitamins is that they don't stay in you. You need to boost your body and keep it boosted by taking the right vitamins to keep up your stamina and strength. The best vitamin is Vitamin B. Let's start by looking on how these vitamins will help you.

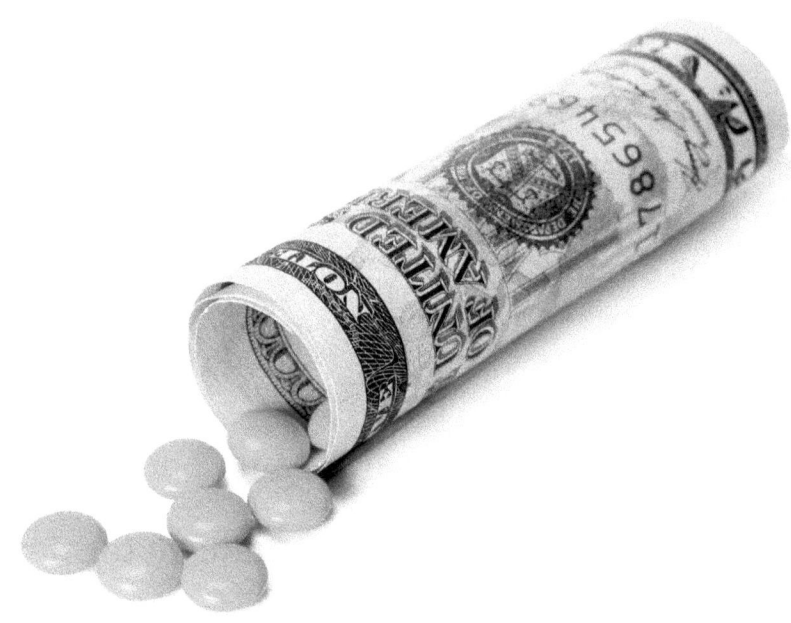

3 B-Vitamins You Can't Live Without

Anyone who has bought health supplements knows how confusing it can be to sift through them. A towering wall of vitamins, minerals, oils, and chemical names greets the average supplement shopper, and it can be dizzying trying to figure out which ones to buy. The **B vitamins** are most confusing of all, since each vitamin is different, but the difference is only denoted by a number. Hopefully this chapter can help to alleviate the consternation by delving into the five major B vitamins and their functions.

Vitamin B-2: Riboflavin

Previously known as the G vitamin, today vitamin B-2 is most commonly known as riboflavin. Touted frequently as a super-nutrient, riboflavin is a key contributor to good health in humans. But just what does riboflavin do exactly?

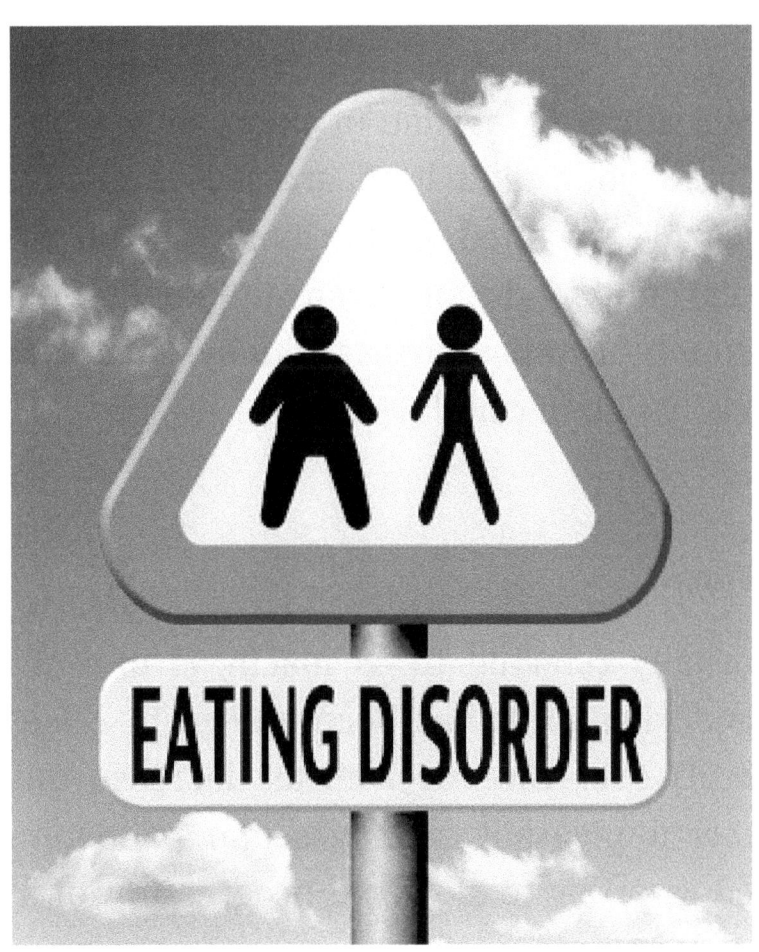

Well, it turns out riboflavin is a key component in many cell processes, most notably those of cell metabolism. It helps cells break down fats, proteins, ketone bodies, and carbohydrates. If you didn't have any riboflavin, your cells would be unable to turn food into energy!

Symptoms of a riboflavin deficiency include inflamed mucus membranes, cracked or sore lips, anemia, sore throat and mouth ulcers. Animal tests have shown a riboflavin deficiency to result in stunted growth, fatigue, inability to stand or walk, and eventually even death.

While people in first-world countries almost never exhibit clinical signs of a riboflavin deficiency, some 28 million Americans are said to suffer from lesser symptoms.

If you're worried about being one of them, or you just want to add some riboflavin to your diet, here are a few good sources. Many processed foods are fortified with riboflavin, such as milk, juice, breakfast cereals, baby foods, and even some energy drinks. It occurs naturally in almonds, legumes, cheese, kidneys, livers, and yeast. Yeast extract is especially rich in riboflavin.

Vitamin B-3: Niacin

Vitamin B-3, usually referred to as niacin, is one of the necessary nutrients for good health. It has been shown to raise levels of HDL (good cholesterol) over time as well as decrease the risk of heart attacks and other unpleasant cardiovascular happenings. It has long been prescribed in order to slow the progression of atherosclerosis, and it can also help to reduce inflammation of veins and arteries.

A deficiency of niacin can manifest primarily in an affliction of pellagra, and nasty skin disease that can also cause dementia. Minor deficiencies can cause a slower metabolism and higher sensitivity to cold. While somewhat rare, deficiencies can appear in first world countries as a side effect of poverty, alcoholism, or malnutrition. You may also be deficient in niacin if you consume corn as a staple food, since corn requires extra processing for its niacin to become available in digestion.

Fortunately, there are many common foods that contain niacin, so a deficiency is easy to avoid. Consuming fish, poultry, beef, eggs, carrots, avocados, tomatoes, broccoli, mushrooms, nuts, and even energy drinks can boost niacin levels. Even a nice cold beer can help fight the good fight against a deficiency, so now you can crack one open guilt-free.

Be careful though, niacin can cause skin irritation and exacerbate conditions like eczema if over-consumed. If you worry you may be consuming too much niacin, talk to your doctor or nutritionist.

Vitamin B-9: Folic Acid

Though it has been called many names, such as Vitamin M and folacin, Vitamin B-9 is most famously called folic acid. Folic acid, usually consumed in the form of folate, can help to reduce the risk of stroke, some forms of cancer, and certain birth defects in children. Taking folate during pregnancy can especially lower the risk of heart defects. It is also necessary for the production of sperm in men.

A folic acid deficiency can lead to birth defects, especially heart defects, as well as sub- or infertility in men and a greater risk of cancer and stroke. Side effects of a deficiency include anemia, weakness, nerve damage, and numbness in certain parts of the body. Fortunately, folic acid stores will take months to run out after intake of folate has stopped, so there is always time to correct one's intake.

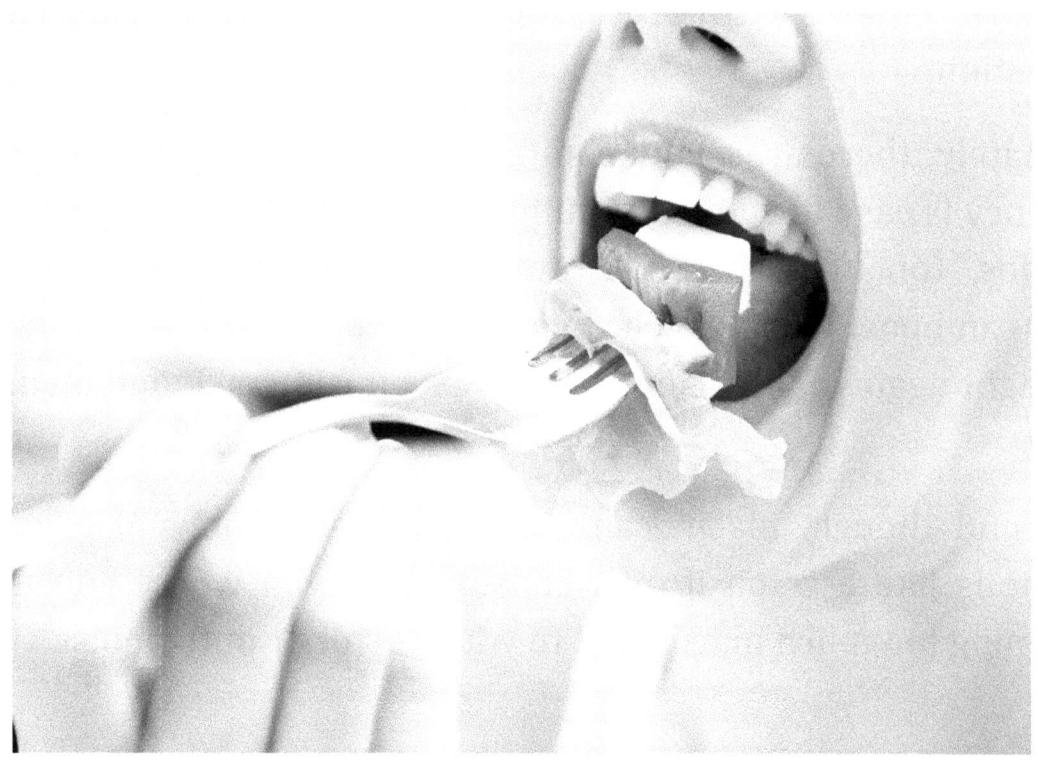

Leafy vegetables are especially good sources of folic acid, which is named after the Latin for "leaf." It can also be found in nuts, beans, peas, seafood, yeast, liver, and even some beers. Spinach, brussel sprouts, and asparagus are some of the best sources for folic acid. Some countries also fortify their processed grains with this essential vitamin.

Be careful: though it is difficult to take a toxic amount of folic acid, some professionals suspect it may worsen the effects of malaria in small children.

Riboflavin, niacin, and folic acid - or vitamins B-2, B-3, and B-9 respectively - are just a few of the essential nutrients your body needs to thrive. Without them, you may find yourself falling apart pretty fast! Hopefully this chapter has made it a little easier to find the ones you need on your next trip to the pharmacy.

3 Start Eating More Fruit : The Best Start to Your New Diet

...

So you have started to use antioxidants and have boosted your strength and stamina with some well needed vitamins. These are the two critical steps to getting your sugar detox on. So it's time to start consuming a natural sugar diet. So eating fruits is the best way. So why fruits you might ask?

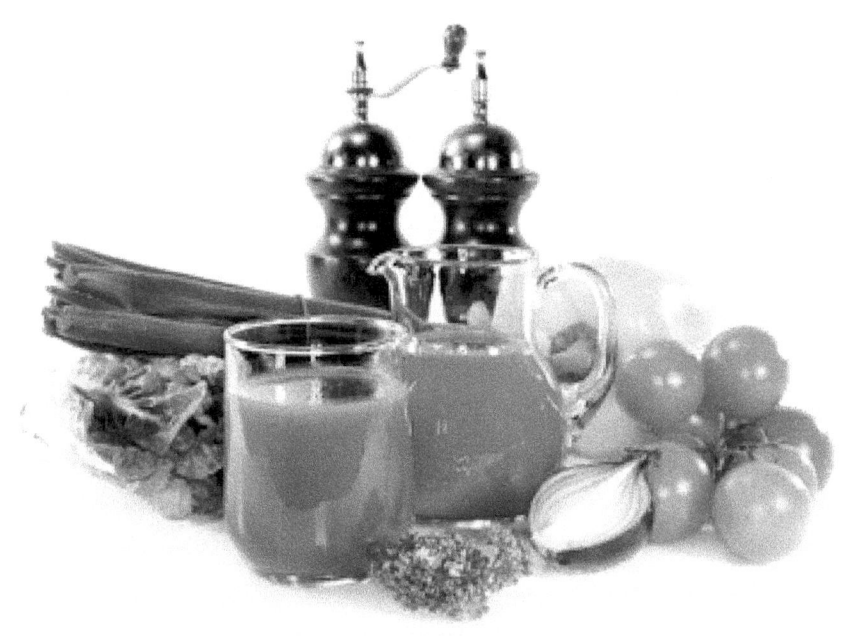

Most people know that they should eat more fruit, but only about 1/3 of Americans actually eat the recommended two to three servings per day. Increasing your fruit intake can have a number of positive effects on your health including decreasing your chance for chronic disease, maintaining healthy blood pressure and providing proper nutrients for healthy eye function. And unlike vegetables, fruits are sweet and delicious, making them much easier to willingly fit into your diet.

The first thing to do when attempting to change your diet is to first assess what is already a part of your diet. A food journal can be an excellent way to truthfully observe what you eat every day. If you happen to find that you are eating at least two to three servings of fruit per day, then there's no need to change your diet.

However, if you are like 2/3 of Americans who don't get their recommended daily serving, there are a couple of simple ways you can increase your fruit intake and reap the benefits of better health.

Adding fruit to your breakfast is one of the simplest ways to increase the amount of fruit in your diet. Whether you choose to eat a whole piece of fruit on the go, or add it to your regular breakfast routine, fruit can be a great morning energy booster.

If you eat cereal every morning, add a whole sliced banana or a handful of blueberries to make a sweet treat even sweeter by getting one whole serving of fruit.

Smoothies are also a great way to get at least one serving of fruit. All you need is a blender and your favorite fruits. You can add milk or yogurt for a creamy texture, or honey for some natural, added sweetness. A bit of ice in your smoothie will keep it chilled the whole way to the office.

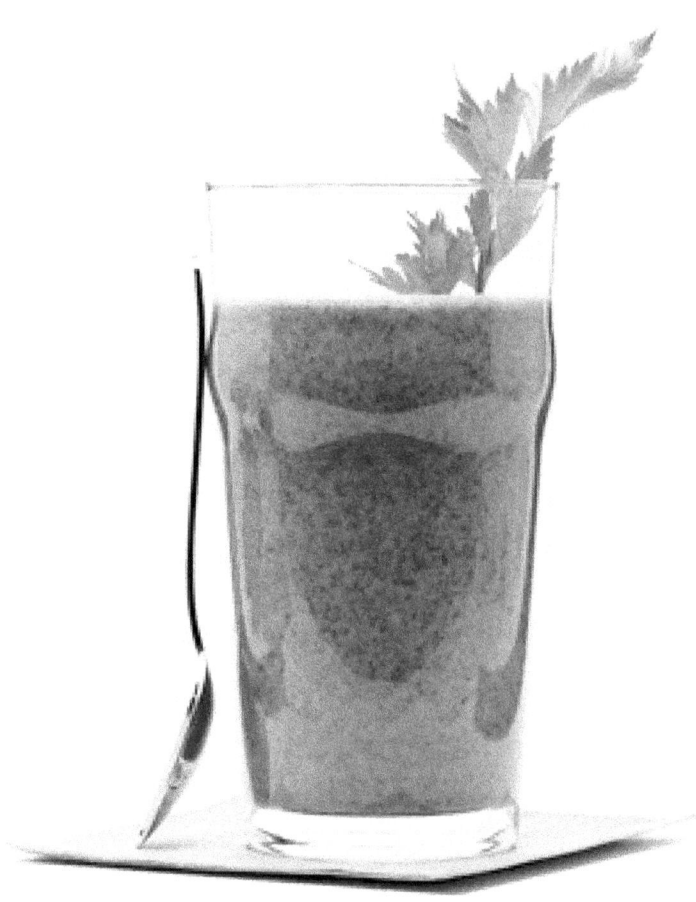

And if you don't have time for these options before work, grabbing an apple, banana or plum on the go is a great way to get something (healthy!) in your stomach when time is limited. Of course, adding a glass of 100% fruit juice to any of these options could fulfill your daily serving in one meal!

Lunchtime can also be a good time to add more fruit to your diet, depending on what you eat for lunch. It's pretty simple to add fruit to salads and sandwiches although the idea might be a little foreign at first. Blueberries go great with tangy dressings and leafy green veggies.

They go especially well with salads with nuts. Sliced apple tastes great with light, crisp salads and sweet dressing. Grapes and oranges are also a good addition to summer salads, and you often don't need much dressing since these fruit are so sweet. If you're more of a sandwich person, sliced fruit can add a bit of flavor to almost any type of sandwich.

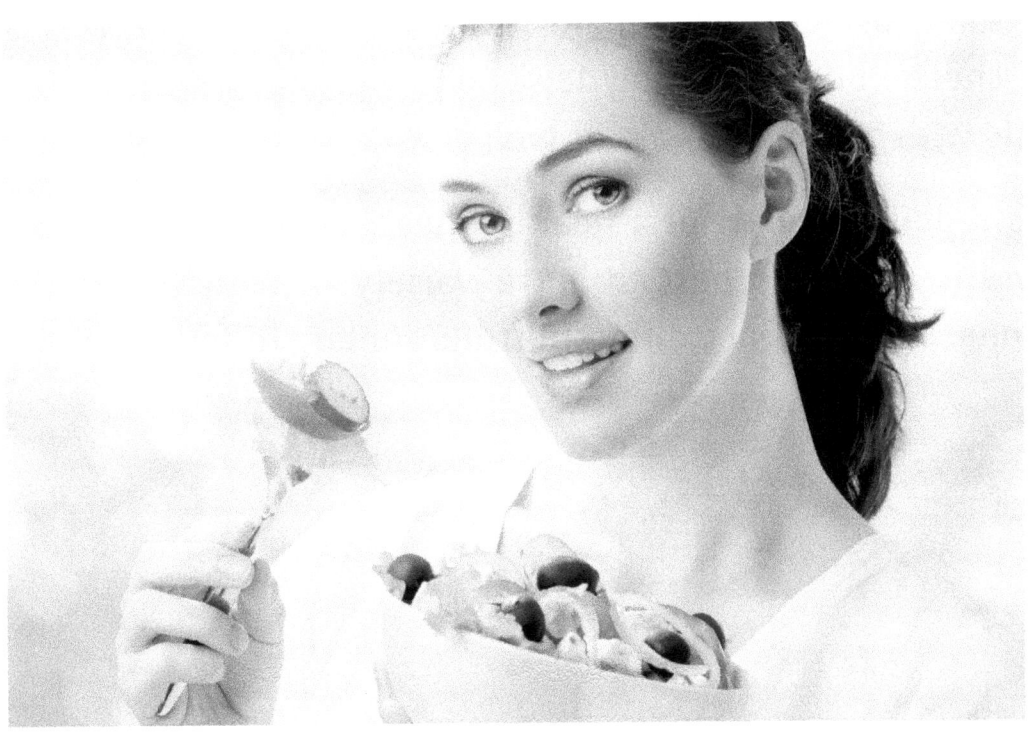

Sliced apples fit nicely with sandwiches that have melted cheese, especially brie and other light cheeses. Bananas taste fantastic between two slices of bread slathered in peanut butter. Add a bit of honey for an extra sweet treat. Although it's a little less practical, a juicy pineapple ring can make a tropical treat out of a ham sandwich or a burger. And remember – tomatoes are fruits, too!

If you're still lacking fruit in your diet by the end of the day, a small dessert or after-dinner snack can often be all you need to fulfill your required daily value. Fruit is inherently sweet, so you can easily satisfy your sweet tooth with a serving of fruit. One of the most healthy, fruity desserts is to simply add a bit of whipped cream to your fruit of choice.

Make sure you go for a light whipped cream, and dunk away. Whipped cream has fewer calories than most other traditional dessert items, and the creaminess will make you feel as though you're getting a treat rather than just grazing on the healthy stuff. Strawberries are the classic choice, but ripe honeydew, purple grapes and peaches all go fantastic with whipped cream as well.

Fruit is a delicious part of a healthy diet that can easily be added to almost any meal. It's best to eat a variety of fruit to get the most nutritional benefits since different fruits contain different nutrients.

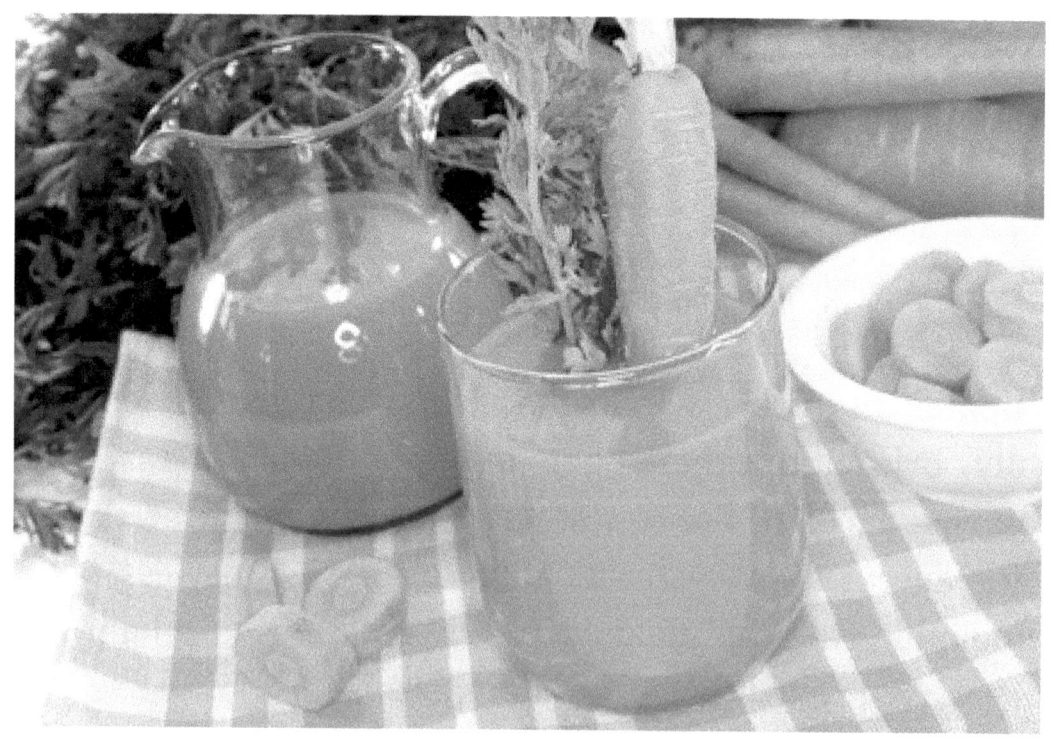

With a bit of meal preparation, you can enjoy the health and taste benefits of a diet rich in fruits.

A good way to add fruit and help with cravings is to keep a bag of dried fruit with you. Just keep an eye on the calories. I know I can eat a whole bag of dried apricots and while they say you can never eat too much fruit, a whole bag of those would back some serious calories!

4 Boosting Your Diet with Superfoods : Forget That Sugar!

. . .

So now you have covered the first three steps it's now time to get into the proper eating regime. Stay away from junk food! You need to start eating specific superfoods that can cleanse you and more importantly the foods that will not topple that sugar cart you call your body!

Cabbage, maple syrup, lemon juice, and rice. What do these things have in common? All are key ingredients in "superfood" diets--fad and crash diets that capitalize on the wondrous, magical properties of one food or food group to stimulate weight loss. But many new fad diets that have desperate dieters storming to grocery stores to stock up on specific foodstuffs are actually past decades' news. Let's take a look at some of the more popular superfoods of yore.

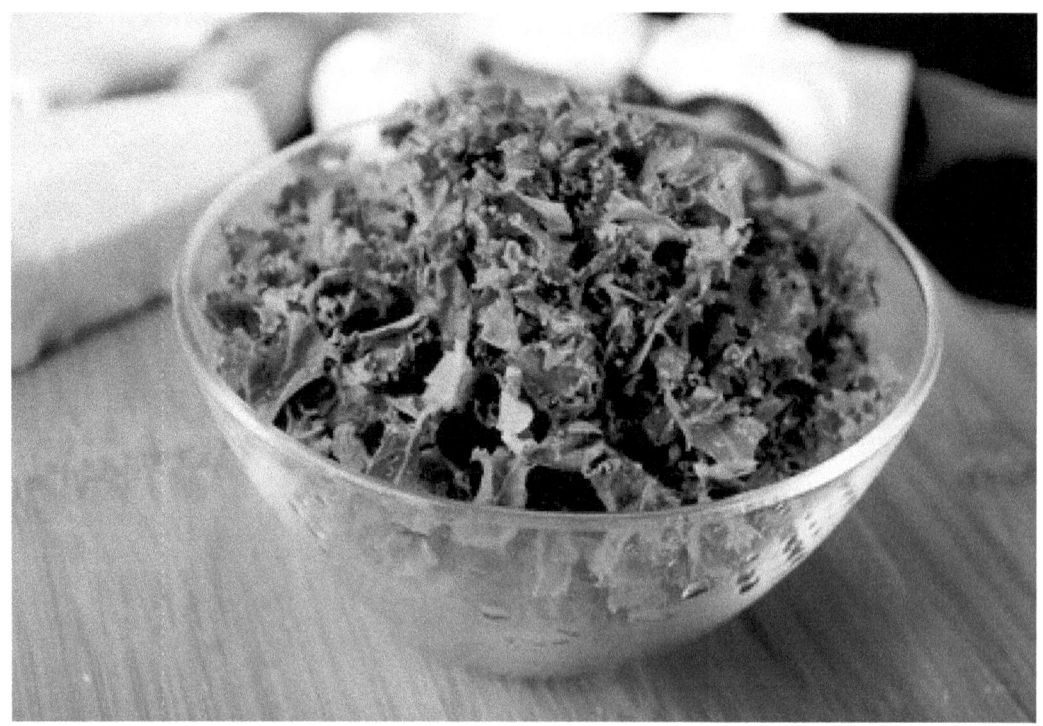

In the 1820s, poet Lord Byron made drinking vinegar and water popular among the haute monde of his time. Byron, who was anorexic and bulimic, already had peculiar dietary habits, which purportedly included stirring a raw egg into his cup of morning tea.

In the 1950's, vinegar made a resurgence when Vermont country doctor D. C. Jarvis incorporated it into the homespun wisdom of his book Folk Medicine, which claimed that ingesting a few teaspoons of vinegar before meals caused food to break down quicker in the gullet.

Although there is no evidence to indicate that vinegar causes weight loss, vinegar diets continue to be popular, as evidenced by numerous websites promoting the Apple Cider Vinegar Diet in its various incarnations.

More recently, retailers have started selling cider vinegar in tablet form--because it takes more than a spoon full of sugar to make this particular "medicine" go down.

It was 1950, the dawning of the atomic age when the Cabbage Soup Diet mysteriously infiltrated the suburban neighborhoods of housewives whose bellies were bloated from canned pseudo-dairies and all those Campbell's "Cream Of" items.

After a 35-year hiatus, instructions for the diet started squeaking through company fax machines under various names, sometimes the Cabbage Soup Diet, other times the Sacred Heart Hospital Diet and even the Mayo Clinic Diet (the clinic categorically denies ownership). By 1990, cabbage soup was once again de rigueur.

The Cabbage Soup Diet involves a confusing seven-day regime in which dieters eat all the cabbage soup they want, as well as very specific foods that could have been drawn from a hat- one day it might be only bananas, the next day a 10-ounce steak. While the exact efficacy of the Cabbage Soup Diet is unknown, it no doubt accounted for a spike in the sale of Gas-X in the early 1990's.

For dieters who can't quite quell their cravings for comfort food, there's always the Rice Diet. This diet was the brainchild of German doctor Walter Kempner, who was a member of Duke University's Department of Medicine in the mid-1930. Kempner made note that people who ate a bowl of white rice every day were less prone to high blood pressure and diabetes and obesity.

Ergo, he developed the rice diet as part of a four-week 1939 boot-camp program in which participants' oral intake was carefully monitored.

Due to it never having been thorough peer review, the Rice Diet languished in fad diet purgatory until 2005, when nutritionist Kitty Rosati and her cardiologist husband, Robert Rosati, dusted off the gauntlet and wrote The Rice Diet Solution based on Kempner's original program.

The no-fat, no-sodium diet, which of course incorporates cooked rice as the main dish of each meal, starts dieters at 800 daily calories and caps them at a lifetime maintenance of 1200--the recommended daily caloric intake for a three-year-old child. However, unlike most superfood diets, The Rice Diet does underscore the necessity of exercise as a key ingredient to the diet's "success."

The crown jewel of superfood diets is the Master Cleanse, aka, the Maple Syrup Diet, aka the Lemonade Diet. Self-professed healer Stanley Burroughs popularized the diet in his book The Master Cleanser, first published in the 1950s. In 2004--when copyright to the *'The Master Cleanser'* would have fallen into public domain, Peter Glickman penned Lose Weight, Have More Energy and Be Happier in 10 Days, which incorporated Burroughs' "cleanse" almost down to the letter.

The diet has dieters consuming exhaustive amounts of water lightly flavored with maple syrup, lemon juice and cayenne pepper.

But the diet's dodgiest procedure is the salt water cleanse, which involves chugging water laden with sea salt to move the bowels along, which also sends dieters howling to the bathroom after the process.

While experts agree that it's possible to lose copious amounts of weight by drinking only sugar and salt water, wilder claims that the diet "cleanses" the body of toxins, curtails alcohol and drug addiction, and increases sexual libido have been debunked.

In 1984, the diet's original creator was charged with second-degree murder for botched treatment of a terminal cancer patient. In addition to administering his infamous diet, Burroughs engaged in medical quackery at its finest to include casting light on the patient using colored stage gels and a common table lamp. Is this the kind of guy you'd trust at your dinner table?

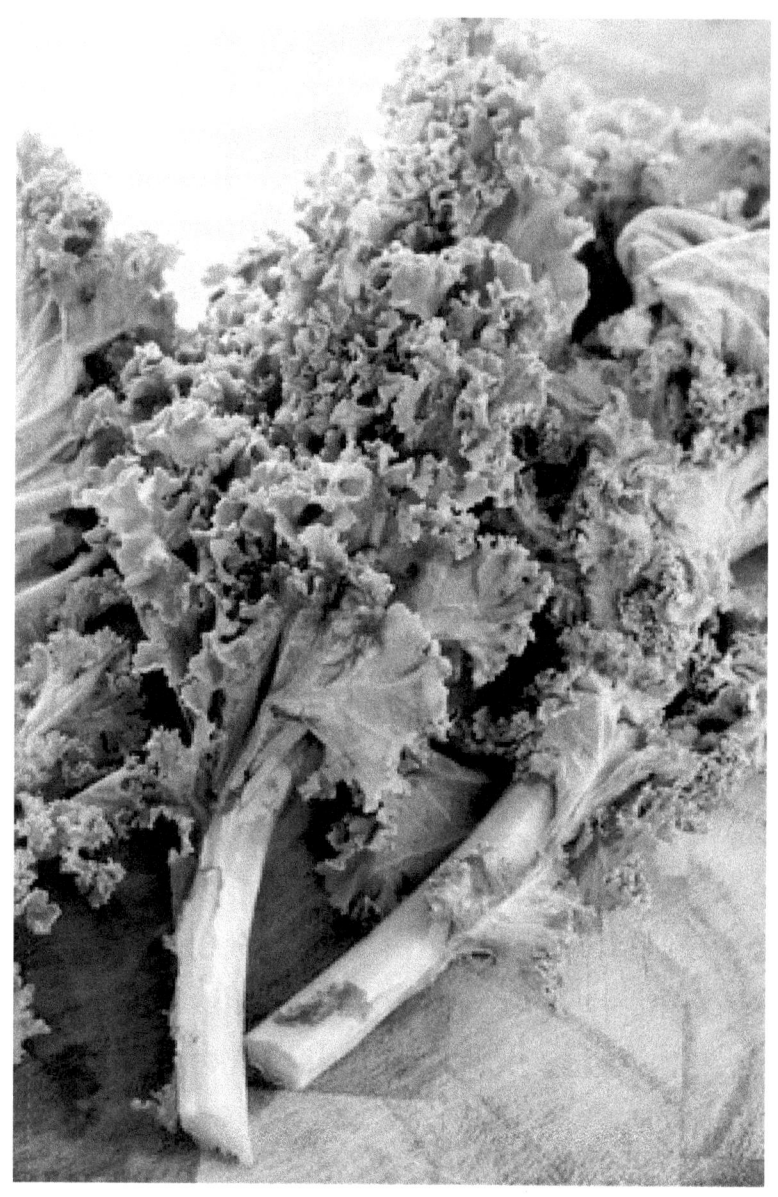

As you can see, many the superfoods of the present are nothing but recycled concepts snagged from the annals of fad diet history. How can you recognize a superfood diet? It's easy. The diet touts one or two foods as a "miracle cure." It ensures rapid, effortless weight loss. It rarely promotes exercise as a component of the diet plan. But what is the hallmark trait of a superfood diet? You won't be able to stay on it for very long and you are usually starving!

A couple easy tips for when you really start to crave something sweet, keep some sugar free gum close by and chew a piece to get your mind off it. Getting up from your chair and just taking a short walk will also help take your mind off it, as long as you don't stroll past a donut shop! And if you do indulge it is not the end of the world, just try to make it a small amount. I learned a trick a while back from a diet specialist.

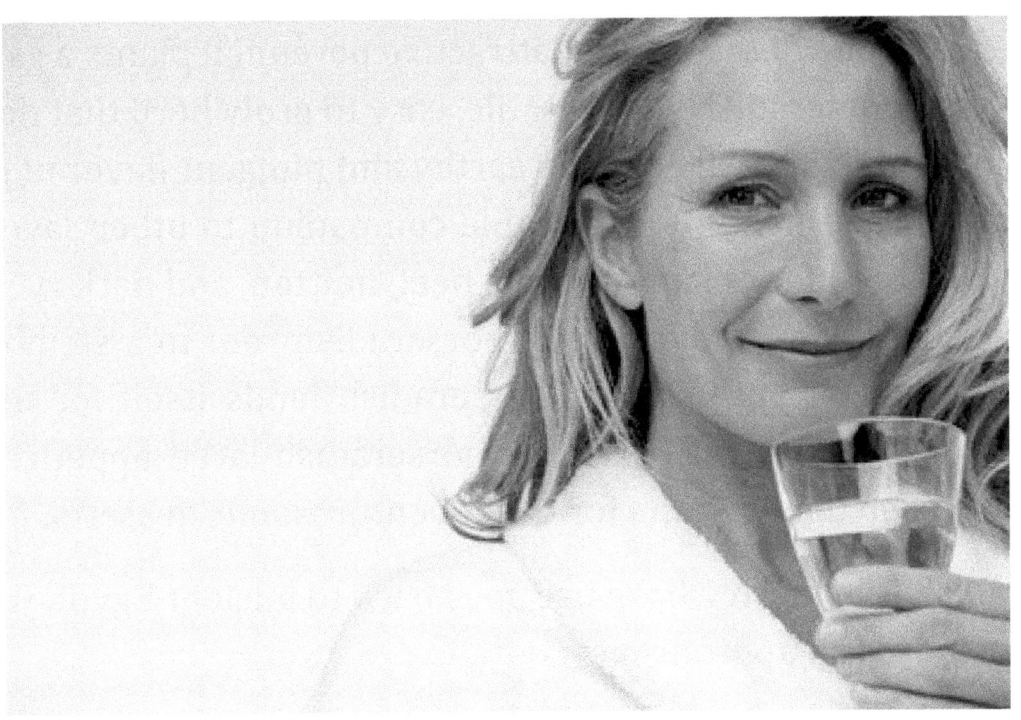

She said to take what you were indulging in, put it on a nice plate and take it to a table and sit down. Then cut it up and eat it with a fork. That way it becomes more of an event and not a quick snack grab. Having to put more thought into it also makes you more aware of what you are doing and cuts back on mindless snacking.

5 Do Not Hold The Horses!

...

One secret weapon I use to tone down on my sugar intake is Horse Radish. There are so many uses of horse radish especially in helping to balance your diet.

Despite being one of the most unattractive perennial plants a gardener can possess, horseradish is a versatile, easy to grow herb that deserves a place in the kitchen garden. The earthy and pungent flavor of ground horseradish root makes it an amiable companion to other savory and strongly flavored foods such as roast beef, mutton, and dark rye bread. Some Germans even add a slice of horseradish root to a stein of beer for a little added zip. In short, horseradish lends itself for use in a plethora of foods; recipes exist for horseradish-laced appetizers and cocktails, roasted meats, and for the adventuresome, desserts.

Horseradish is an herb whose use goes back to ancient Egypt, where it was considered an aphrodisiac.

Later in time, Greek and Roman athletes used horseradish-infused olive oil as a pain reliever for sore muscles. As trade became more global, western European cultures became acquainted with the herb, and embraced it as part of their catalog of culinary condiments. By the 1600s, horseradish was an element in kitchen gardens throughout eastern and western Europe.

Although the medicinal value of horseradish may be greatly exaggerated, it does have some antibacterial properties. Food scientists at Oklahoma State University discovered that the isothiocyanate in horseradish deters the growth of Listeria, E. coli and

Staphylococcus aureus bacteria. Apparently, these food-borne pathogens don't like it hot.

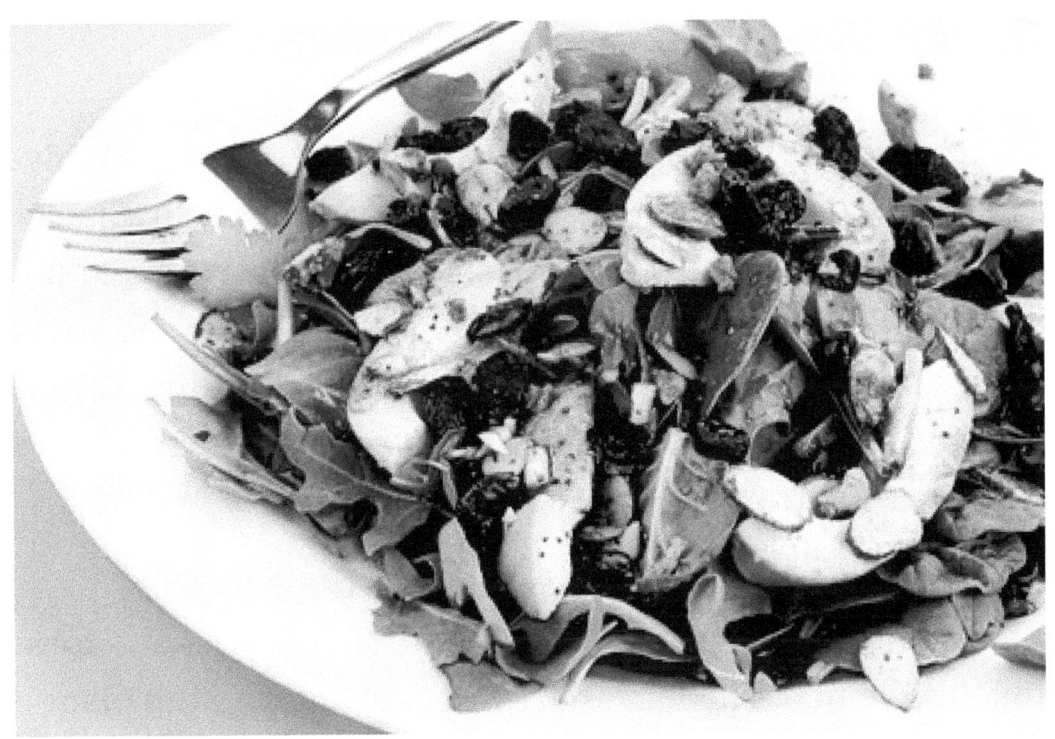

The horseradish capital of North America is Collinsville, Illinois. Located on the banks of the Mississippi River, Collinsville is blessed with potash-rich (an alkaline potassium compound) river bottom soil, cold winters and a long growing season, all of which are nirvana to the horseradish plant.

Like most root crops, horseradish appreciates nutrient rich soil with roughly equal proportions of sand, silt, and clay.

Light, well drained soils allow the root to expand and grow uniformly. However, horseradish tolerates mucky clay. As long as the soil doesn't bake into a substance reminiscent of adobe, horseradish will thrive. The roots may be a little misshapen, but the flavor stays intact.

Horseradish is a perennial plant in USDA zones 5 through 9; north of zone 5, it is best treated as an annual, and roots should be replanted in early spring. The roots, or crowns, should be planted three inches below the surface in soil that has been well loosened and has been enriched with potash.

Organic gardeners who own wood burning stoves have an advantage here, as aged wood ash is an excellent source of potash. Space plants two to three feet apart; happy horseradish plants can have top growth that reaches 30 inches in height and a foot in width. The roots grow downward and expand in equal proportion to the tops. Horseradish likes full sun, and benefits from a light mulch of grass clippings, chopped leaves or straw.

This helps to keep the bed weed-free and the soil from drying out completely, which allows the root to fatten up without forking or becoming misshapen. The leaves are large, ovoid, and the plant itself is generally homely, so keeping the horseradish bed toward the back may help preserve the aesthetics of the garden bed.

Roots are harvested in either fall or spring, and after a good growing cycle may take some muscle to bring out of the ground in one piece. Using a sharp spade, cut a circle around the plant that is at least twelve inches deep all the way around. Plunge the blade of the spade in as deeply as it can go, and then rock the root upward.

Wash the excess dirt off with a garden hose before trimming off the tops. The root resembles a gargantuan version of its cousin, the White Icicle radish. If any part of the root breaks off, it will restart growth and become next year's harvest. The bed may expand from a few plants to a multitude with little effort on the part of the gardener.

Before storing the freshly dug roots, use a vegetable brush or nylon scrubber to wash off any dirt that adheres to the small crevices in the outside skin of the root. Refrigerate fresh horseradish with its skin on in a tightly sealed plastic bag. This helps to retain flavor, and keeps the rather pervasive odor from penetrating other foods. If the root is to be frozen, peel it before bagging.

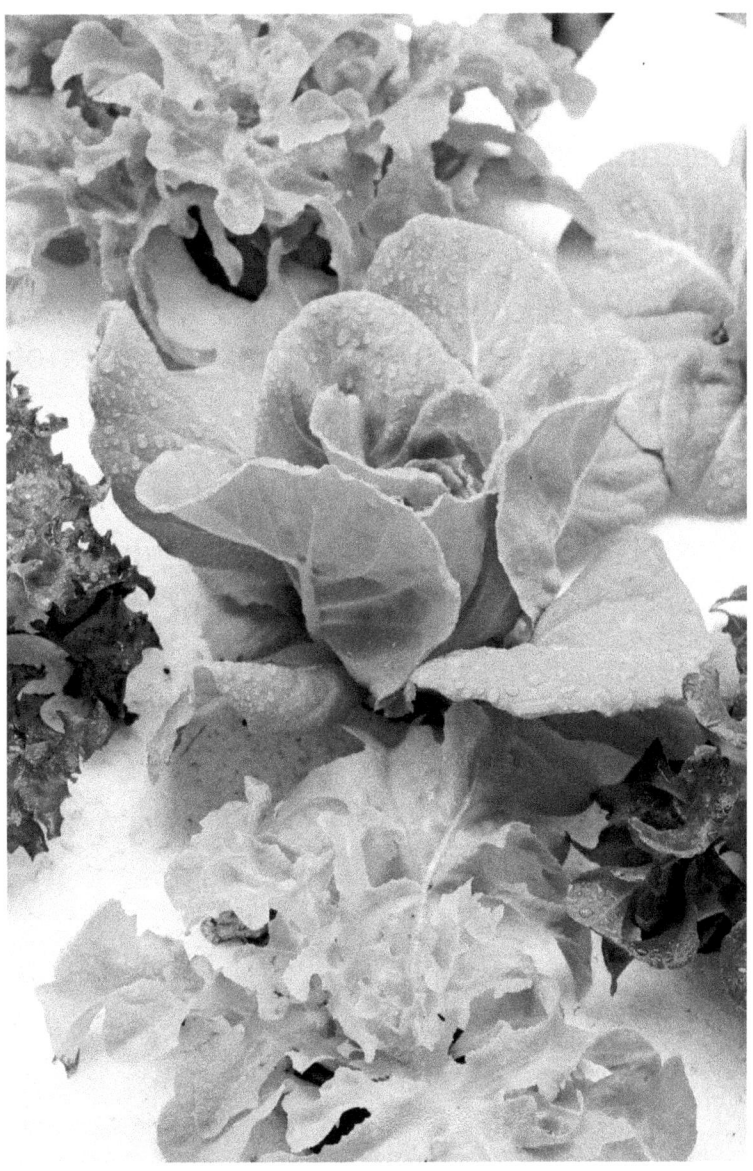

When the cells of the horseradish root are bruised or crushed, it starts a chemical reaction within the cell walls that makes the horseradish hot. Vinegar, lemon, lime or tomato juice stops the reaction, so chopping horseradish root with any of these acids or a (product containing them, such as mayonnaise or hollandaise sauce) will create a very mild condiment.

For full-blown horseradish heat, allow the chopped or grated horseradish to seep in its own juices for a while before adding vinegar, lemon juice, sour cream or mayonnaise. A word of caution: horseradish tarnishes silver, so serve any product containing horseradish with stainless steel implements from a glass container.

What dishes benefit from the addition of horseradish? Try adding a few tablespoons of grated horseradish root and a cup of shredded Cheddar cheese to two cups of creamy mashed potatoes. Sliver some horseradish root into a batch of pickled beets or kosher dill pickles.

Cranberry conserve with horseradish added becomes a sweet, hot, tart topper for all of that leftover turkey from Thanksgiving. As for using horseradish in dessert dishes, the Horseradish Information Council (yes, there really is an advocacy group for horseradish) offers several recipes on their website that are worth trying.

6 Coffee, Coffee and Coffee!

...

When I feel for something sugary – do you know what I have? That's right a cup of coffee. One of the best ways to beat sugar addiction is with a cup of coffee. Try not to have more than one to two cups per day. However the great thing about coffee is that not only does it help to curb your sugar cravings but it has so many other great benefits.

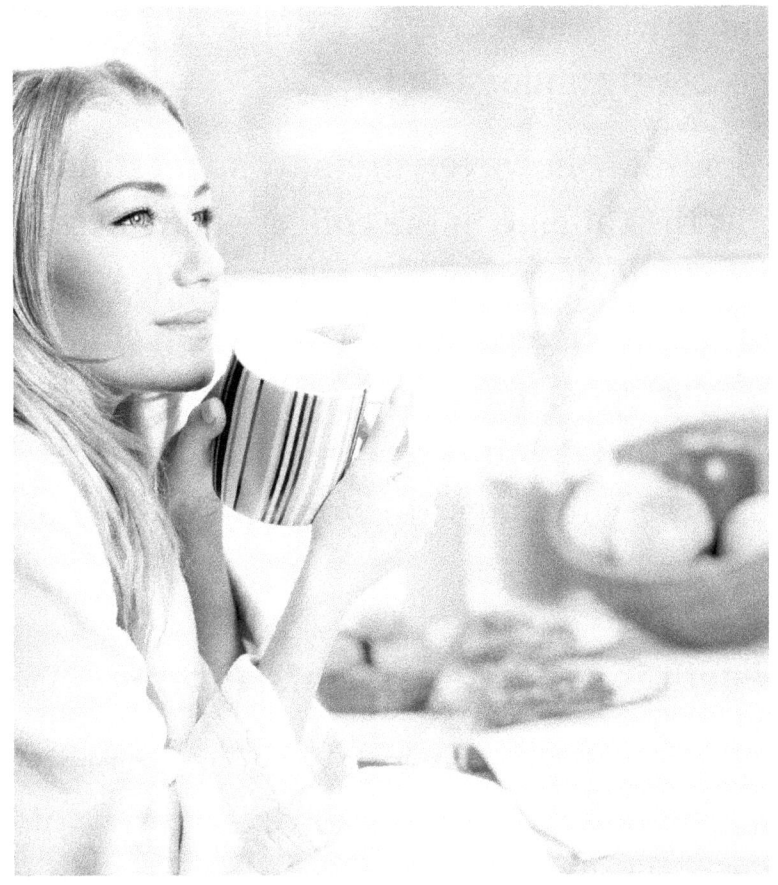

In fact for many people, a morning without coffee is only slightly less excruciating than being hanged, drawn and quartered. The prospect of forswearing coffee entirely is inconceivable. Fortunately, you can now indulge in your morning cup of Joe without guilt; recent studies have suggested that it may have unexpected health benefits. Let us explore some of those here.

The first benefit is that it can reduce the risk of Diabetes.

Multiple studies have shown a correlation between coffee consumption and lower rates of type 2 diabetes, but until recently the relationship was poorly understood.

Researchers from UCLA, however, are now suggesting that coffee—or, more specifically, the caffeine in the coffee—may increase blood levels of a protein that regulates sex hormones like testosterone and estrogen, which have been linked to the development of type 2 diabetes. Given that type 2 diabetes accounts for roughly 90 percent of diabetes cases and can lead to poor circulation, strokes, kidney failure and heart attacks, these findings are worth paying attention to.

The second benefit is a reduced risk of Cancer.

At least among developed countries, cancer is probably the most dreaded of diseases. Coffee drinkers, however, can rejoice; for reasons that are not yet entirely understood, the beverage seems to play a preventative role in the development of some cancers.

For example, researchers at Rutgers recently uncovered a link between increased caffeine consumption and decreased rates of skin cancer- specifically, one 8-ounce cup of coffee per day reduced skin cancer rates by about 5 percent, with higher rates of consumption showing a correspondingly lower risk.

However, it must be noted that where skin cancer in particular is concerned, women appear to benefit disproportionately from the effects of caffeine; a Harvard study found that while women who drank three cups of coffee a day were 20 percent less likely to develop basal cell skin carcinoma, the risk for men who consumed the same amount of caffeine was reduced by only 9 percent.

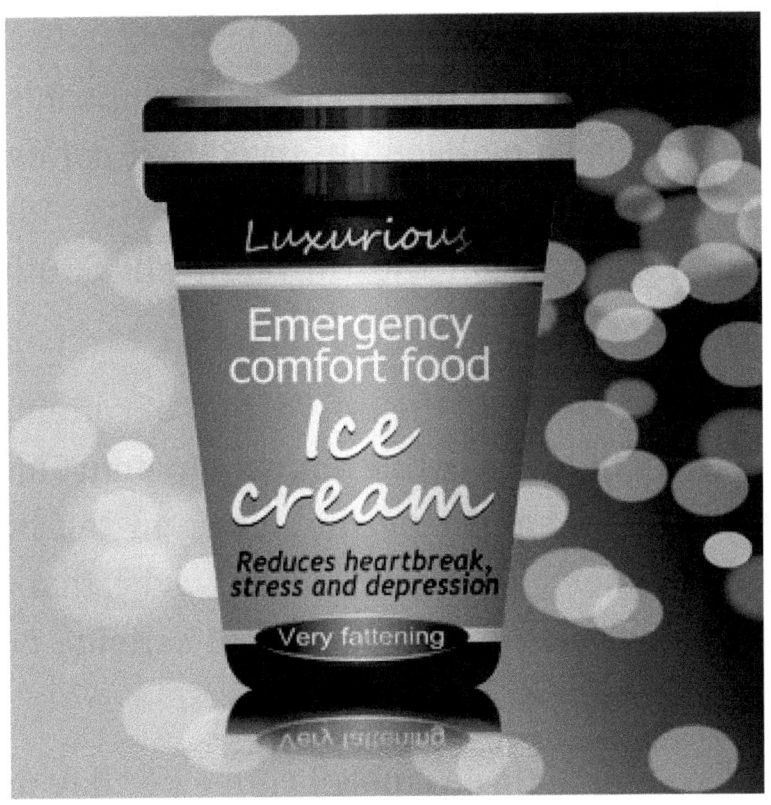

There is, however, good news for men. According to researchers at Harvard, drinking coffee—regular or decaf—was associated with lower rates of aggressive prostate cancer. On the flip side, several studies have suggested that high rates of caffeine consumption in women may moderately reduce the risk of breast cancer, although these findings may apply only to postmenopausal cancers.

Finally, coffee consumption appears to reduce the risk of colorectal cancer, although exactly how effective it is remains uncertain; various studies have found that those who consume the most coffee enjoy a risk reduction of anywhere from 24 to 56 percent.

The third benefit, there appears to be protection against some degenerative diseases.

Coffee may also offer protection against Parkinson's disease and Alzheimer's. While it has long been observed that coffee consumption during middle and old age is associated with lower rates of Alzheimer's, a new study from the University of South Florida may offer some clues as to why.

According to these researchers, the interaction of caffeine and some as yet unknown ingredient in the coffee appears to boost blood levels of a growth factor found at abnormally low levels in the brains of those suffering from Alzheimer's. Bear in mind, however, that these findings apply only to those with a fairly high rate of caffeine consumption—that is, four or more cups per day.

By contrast, a mere two to three cups of coffee per day may be enough to reduce your risk of Parkinson's by 25 to 30 percent. On the other hand, a 2010 study suggests that these benefits may only apply to those who carry a gene that amplifies the effect of the caffeine. Still, given that a quarter of the population is thought to possess this gene, drinking coffee certainly won't hurt you.

Forth benefit, coffee can help protect your liver.

It's always nice when one vice cancels out another. Scientists have known about the link between alcohol consumption and liver damage for years, but what has only recently come to light is the role coffee may play in protecting the liver.

Multiple studies have revealed that the risk of alcohol-related cirrhosis is greatly reduced among coffee drinkers—perhaps by as much as 80 percent in those who drink four or more cups of coffee a day. Moreover, other research suggests that in enjoying their morning pick-me-up, coffee drinkers may be halving their risk of liver cancer.

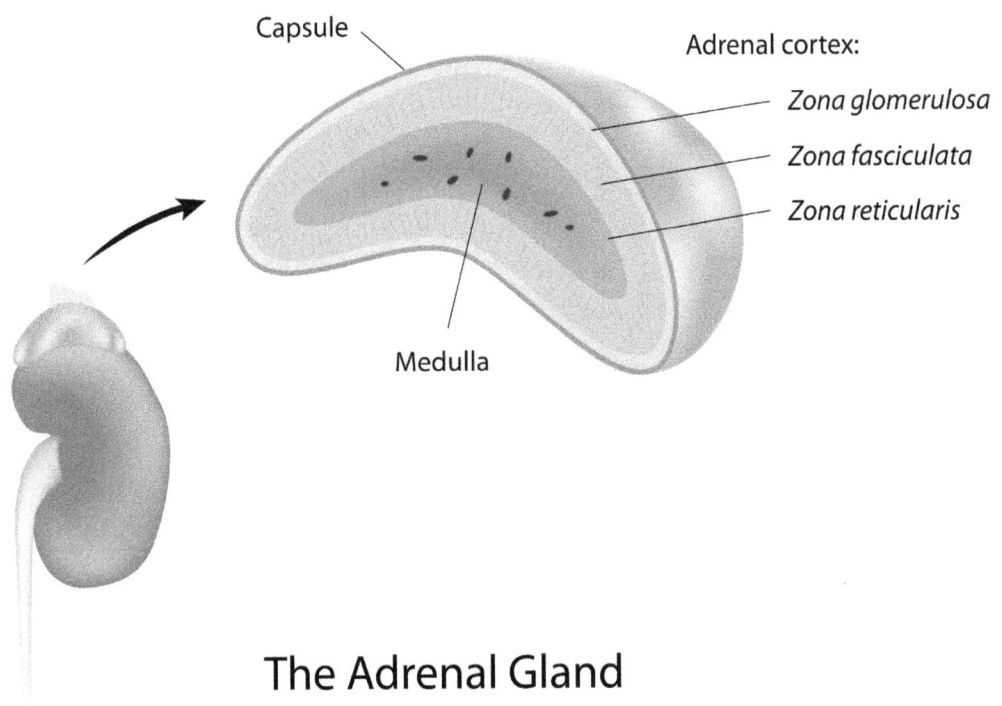

The Adrenal Gland

The fifth benefit, coffee drinkers have a reduced risk of depression.

For all those who feel grumpy when they miss their morning coffee, this one may seem like a no-brainer. However, the focus of this Harvard study is not the run-of-the-mill gloominess we all experience now and then, but rather clinical depression—a serious disease with a lifetime prevalence of roughly 20 percent in the United States.

That the risk of depression was found to be 20 percent lower among coffee drinkers is therefore nothing to sneer at.

Unfortunately, these benefits again appear to be restricted to women, but given that depression is more common in women to begin with, the findings are still significant. Be careful, though—too much caffeine can lead to irritability and even anxiety.

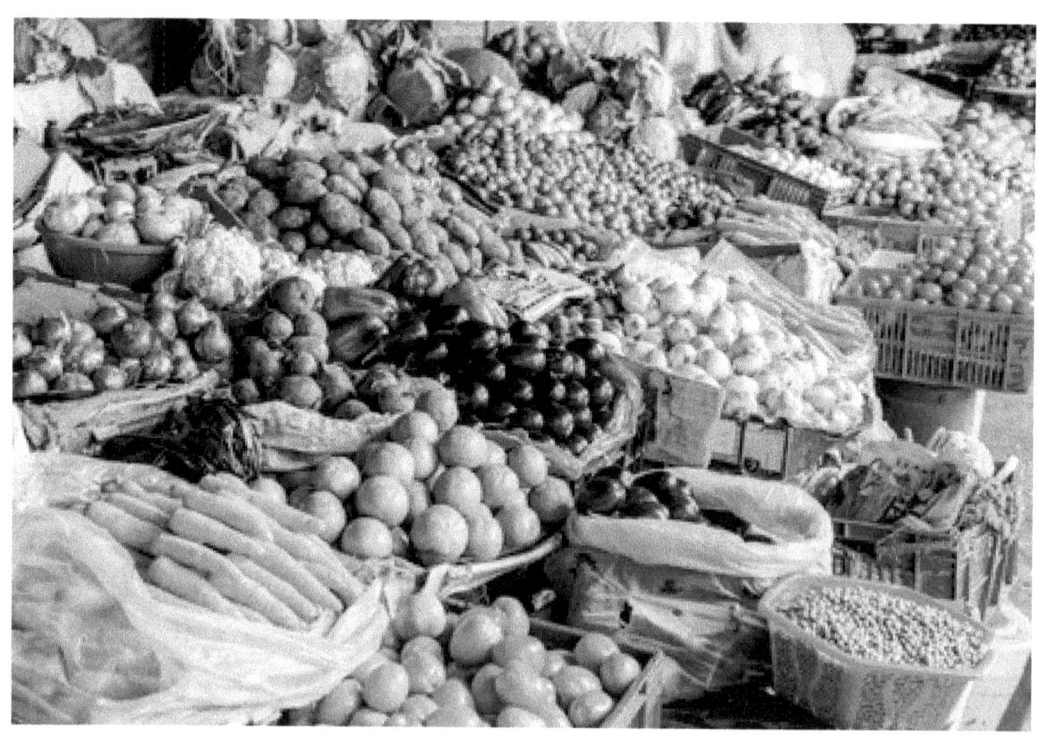

Here is a favorite smoothie mix of mine that soothes my sugar and coffee craving. I usually will mix this up as a mid-day or afternoon pick me up. I call it the Cocoa Caffinator.

Cocoa Caffinator Smoothie

Take one banana, ¼ cup coconut milk, 1 tablespoon of cocoa powder, a teaspoon of almond butter and around 6 coffee ice cubes (you have to think ahead a bit on this one!). You can also use 3 ice cubes and cooled coffee. Mix and enjoy. You will need to experiment with the amounts in this one. I have found everyone seems to like it a bit different but it is good even when it is not perfect!

7 THE SECRET FOODS THAT BUSTS SUGAR

. . .

These are my favorite foods that help to kill my sugar cravings.

Don't forget the powerful health benefits that these foods provide are reason enough to consider adding them to your diet.

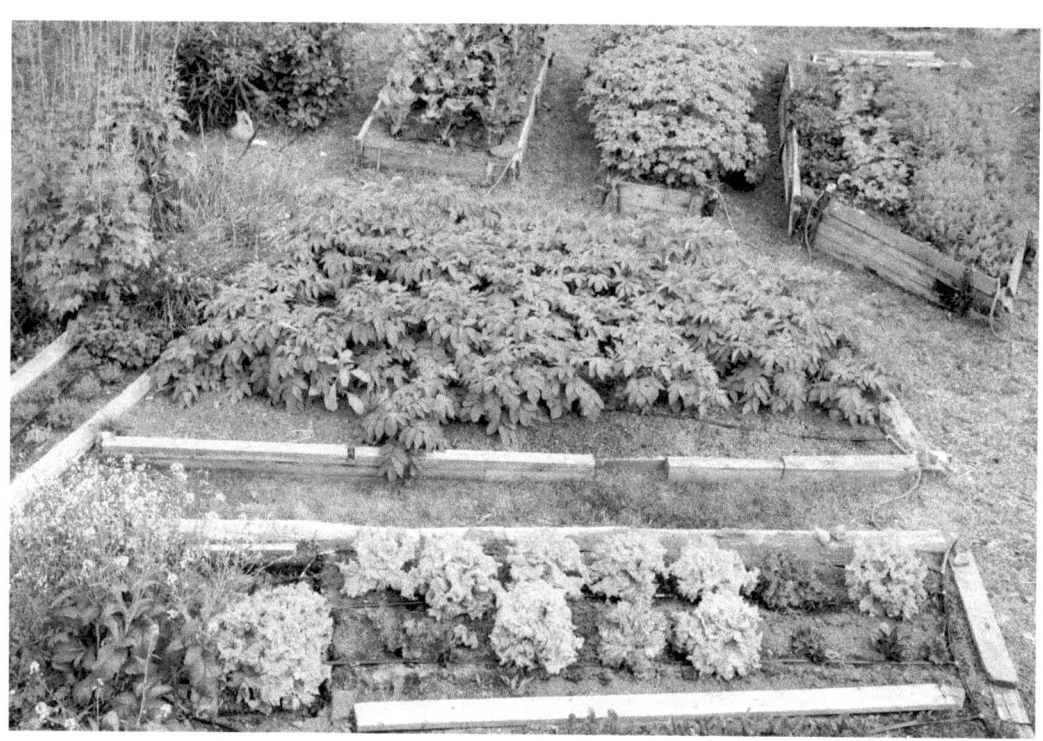

Kimchi (or Kimchee)

Kimchi has been very popular for many years in Korea, but not so much in the United States. Kimchi is made of fermented cabbage or radish, and Koreans eat it with most of their meals.

Kimchi is high in fiber, low in calories, and rich in vitamins A, B, and C. It also has "healthy" bacteria called lactobacilli which are highly beneficial for your digestive system.

The taste of kimchi depends on how it is prepared. Usually it is spicy, and it is typically prepared with a mix of salt, vinegar, garlic, red chili peppers, and other spices.

You don't have to learn how to prepare kimchi (unless you want to). It is sold in some grocery stores and markets.

Calf Liver

Calf liver sounds delicious, right? No, not really. But it is a healthy food that is filled with healthy goodness.

A slice of calf liver provides copious amounts of vitamins A and B and the minerals phosphorus, zinc, copper, and selenium. It is also a low fat meat and excellent protein source.

Calf liver is a bit high in cholesterol, which is why it should be eaten in moderation.

Beef Brains

When you're feeling very hungry and craving food, eating a plate of beef brains is probably the last thing you would think of. But beef brains are popular in France, Italy, Mexico, and other Latin American and European countries.

Beef brain is high in the minerals niacin, phosphorus, selenium, and vitamins C and B12. Unfortunately, beef brains also have lots of cholesterol. The vitamin and mineral content gives beef brains a healthy kick, but you should eat it sparingly due to the cholesterol.

Beef brains are prepared many different ways. They can be made into burgers, blended with eggs, or made into stews or soups. A quick online search will turn up dozens of ways to prepare and season brains to make them tasty.

Wheatgrass

Obviously, wheatgrass does not sound very appetizing, but it is a very healthy superfood.

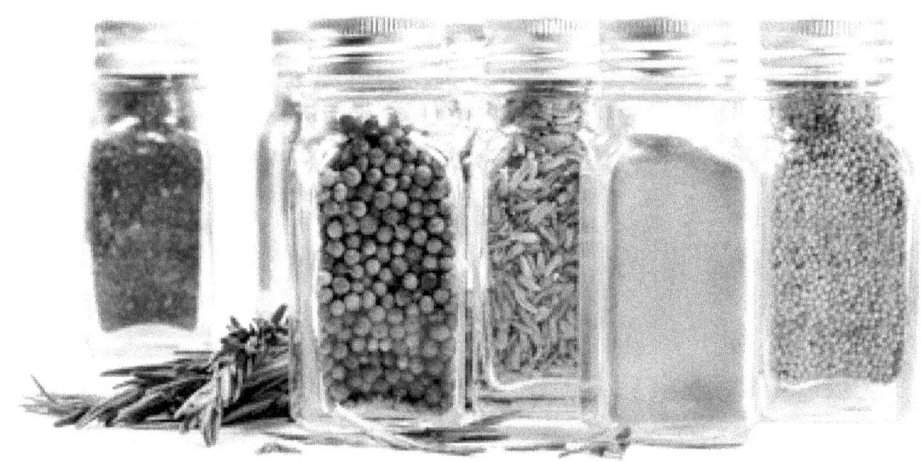

Wheatgrass is full of vitamins and minerals. It's rich in vitamins A, E, K, and B. Wheatgrass packs a powerful health punch that rivals many fruits and vegetables.

Wheatgrass is not considered a tasty health food. However, you can make it palatable by blending it with other ingredients (like fruit) in a shake. Some people prefer to take wheatgrass shots, but you can also buy it in tablet form if you want to bypass the taste of it.

Cod Liver Oil

Cod liver oil is extracted from the liver of the Codfish. The oil is rich in vitamins A, D, and E. It also contains omega-3, a type of fat that is highly important for maintaining good health.

Your body needs the nutrients in cod liver oil to maintain strong bones, healthy skin, strong joints, and more.

The downside is the strong oily taste of liquid cod liver oil. However, the good news is that it is available in pill form, so you don't necessarily have to taste it.

Marmite

Marmite is the brand name for a food spread made from yeast extract. The spread is popular in the U.K., South Africa, Australia and New Zealand. Many vegans and vegetarians use Marmite in the U.S.

Marmite contains high amounts of vitamins in the B group. It's also high in sodium, which is one reason (besides the strong taste) people use it in small amounts.

Marmite tastes salty and bitter, and it's normally used in small amounts as a flavor enhancer. Many enjoy small amounts of the spread on crackers and toast. It can also be used on some vegetables and other food items.

The British and Australian versions of Marmite have distinct tastes, and people either love the spread or they absolutely hate it.

I realize that those six foods don't sound very appetizing, but that shouldn't stop you from giving them a try. With a little experimentation, trial and error, you can make almost any food palatable by preparing it in a way that's pleasing for your taste buds.

8   Get Rid Of The Msg : This Is The Final Tip For Sugar Busting

...

A few years ago Monosodium Glutamate, known as MSG, was called out for being a dangerous food additive, prompting many manufacturers to remove it from their products.

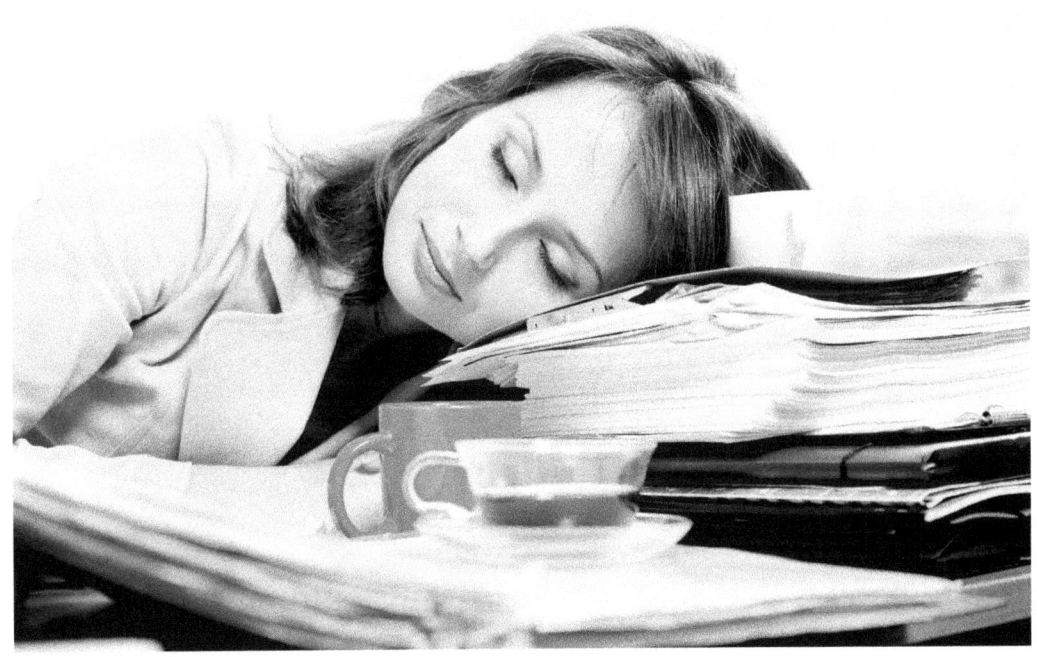

Or so we thought. In reality, MSG continues to be added to our foods in large quantities and often without our knowledge. That's because manufactures have found a way to hide it in food by using dozens of obscure names and they do it all with the approval of the FDA.

Even products that claim to be MSG free often still contain the additive. Legally, manufactures are only required to list MSG if they specifically add it as an ingredient. So, if one of the other listed ingredients contains MSG they do not have to put it on the package.

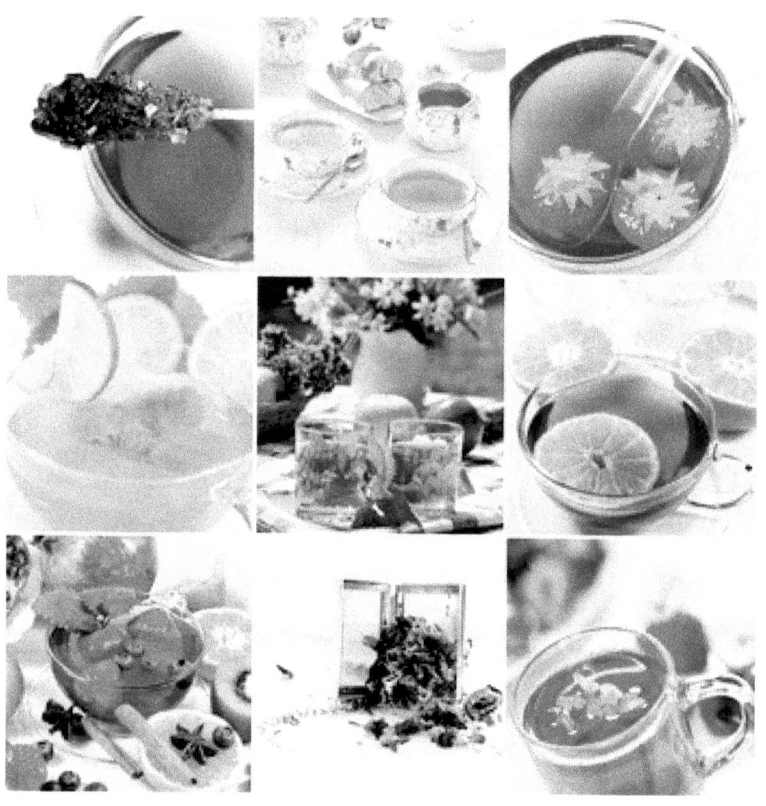

The Dangers of MSG

Studies have shown that MSG causes brain legions in mice and one of the biggest dangers is the devastating affect it may have on the human brain.

MSG has been linked to dozens of issues from simple headaches and bloating to serious health problems such as obesity, autism, neurological disorders, cancer and many other diseases. Unfortunately, for every scientific study showing a link between MSG and disease, food and drug manufactures have their own studies claiming the additive is not harmful to humans.

The FDA appears to sit squarely on the fence in this matter admitting that large quantities of MSG can be harmful but also claiming that the amount in our food is safe for consumption.

The problem with that theory is that MSG is in so many different products that it would be impossible for anyone to know when they have reached an unsafe level.

Finding MSG

You can find MSG hiding in almost every processed food on grocery store shelves including packaged dinners, soups, beans, canned vegetables, spices, and even milk and dairy products. A few manufacturers are honest enough to list MSG or monosodium glutamate on the label but most likely it will be disguised under a different name.

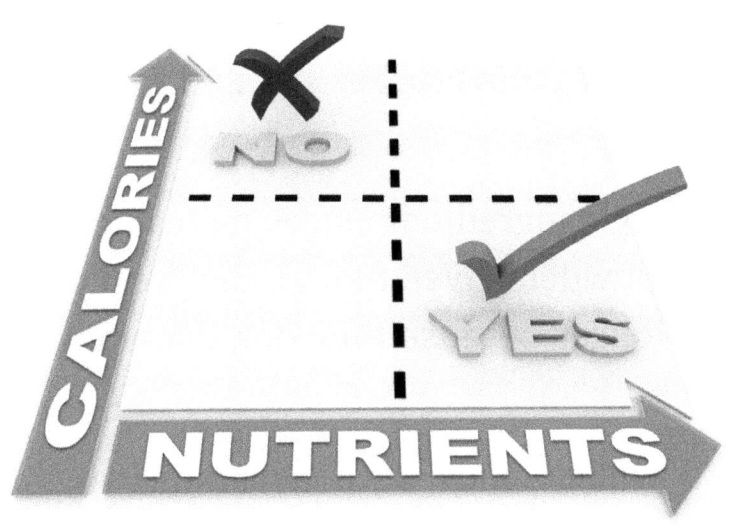

Some of the more common names you might find are Calcium Caseinate, Gelatin, Hydrolyzed products, Soy or Whey Protein and Yeast Nutrient, but there are dozens of others and new names are added all the time. MSG can also be hiding in the deceptively simple form of natural flavorings or spices.

Avoiding MSG

Unless you grow all your own food, eliminating all MSG from your diet may be nearly impossible, but that doesn't mean you can't cut it down to a safer level. Following are some simple ways to quickly reduce the amount of MSG in your diet:

Stay away from all pre-packaged dinners and sauces and switch to whole grain plain pasta with toppings you make yourself from fresh ingredients.

Avoid canned vegetables and opt for frozen ones that are usually more nutritious anyway.

Take canned beans off your grocery list and start making your own using dried beans.

Buy high quality single ingredient spices instead of combination ones such as many chili powders. Even though they're more expensive, they usually last much longer because they don't contain other fillers such as salt or sugar.

Cook with more whole foods such as onions, potatoes and fresh produce.

Choose whole grain bread products that contain fewer ingredients that you can actually understand.

If you're worried about the effects of MSG on your family, then it is time to get serious about controlling the foods you serve.

There are plenty of recipes on the internet and you may be pleasantly surprised to learn that you can cook wholesome and delicious MSG-free meals in about the same amount of time it takes to make a packaged product.

Investing a small amount of money in a crock pot will also make cooking meat, beans, soups and chili a breeze with very little effort on your part.

Switching to a healthier diet will also help you cut down on other dangerous ingredients such as bleached white flour, sugars, hydrogenated products and high fructose corn syrups that are often found in processed foods. The human body has amazing restorative powers but we can't keep feeding it poison without serious or even fatal consequences. Eliminating as much MSG as possible may go a long way in strengthening immune systems and preventing many health issues.

Conclusion

I hope the information contained in my book will help you to make more healthy choices and enable you to start to detox your body of extra and unnecessary sugars, and replace them with healthy foods.

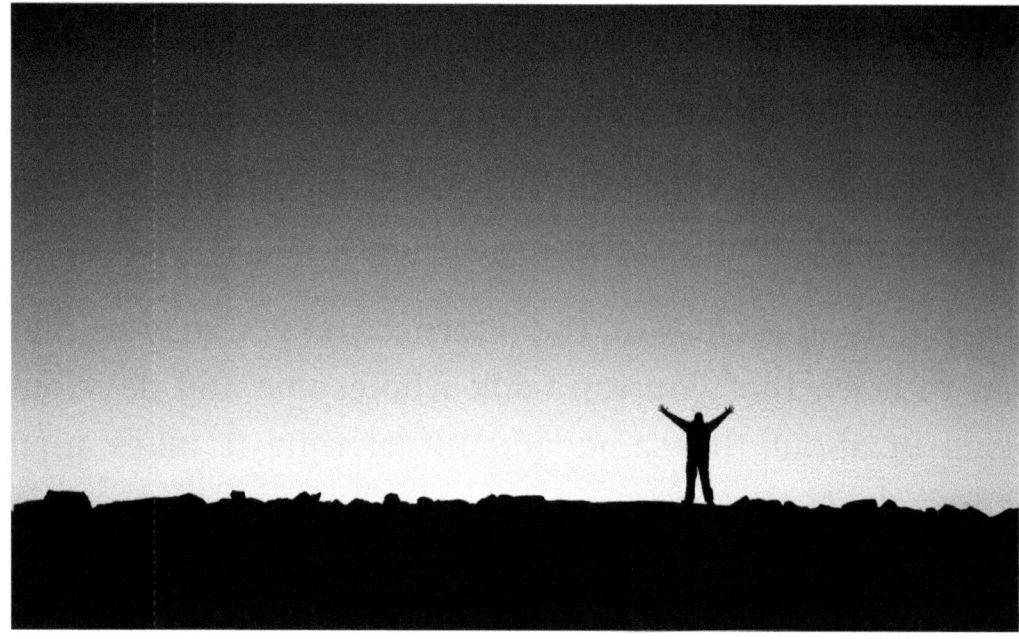

Start slowly if you need to, replace one not so healthy item a day for a week (if you are a tea drinker and enjoy it with milk for instance, use a smaller and smaller amount each day until you eliminate it and you will actually find after a few weeks you won't even like it with milk anymore!) and then the following week swap out another one.

You will start to feel better and better each day and you will find you will crave those unhealthy foods less and less as each day passes. How good you feel is your body thanking you for treating it better!

The Most Important Thing You Can Do To Spread The Word

I thank you for reading my book.

If I may just ask if you could spare me just a few minutes of your precious time, to **LEAVE A REVIEW TODAY** if you have indeed enjoyed reading the stories in this book.

If you could, please help to spread the word around by leaving a review.

WHY REVIEWS MATTER

It is every writer's desire to have their book being held in the hands of readers such as you, and to share in the writer's belief in the stories.

As it is a very competitive environment out there in the publishing world, with many writers wanting to be noticed, asking for reviews is one of the most pragmatic ways we can gain more readers to share in our stories.

It is through getting and reading reviews from you, that writers like me get encouraged and to be spurred in writing more exciting stories to share with all of you.

Will You Be a Part of Our 1%?

The truth of the matter is, many who read a book seldom review it. In fact, less than 1% of them do.

Reasons for not leaving a review are plentiful….

Some say it is too tedious to write.

Some have absolutely no idea what to write.

For some, it never even came cross their mind to review the book.

Or they simply claim it is a waste of their time.

If you truly do not wish to review my book, I totally understand. You have already blessed my heart by reading my book, and I thank you for that.

If however, you choose to belong to that 1% readers who are willing to lend writers a helping hand, to help us get noticed, it will be most ideal.

Indie authors such as us seek audience and it is through word-of-mouth and reviews at Amazon, Apple, Barnes & Nobel, Goodreads, and similar sites that can make all the difference in the world between whether a new reader will find and buy our books.

All I need is just a few minutes and it would have made a **huge difference** in how indie writers' stories will unfold.

Your words need not be long. Just honest words, truthful feedback of the reasons why you enjoyed reading the book and this would mean the world to me.

Please go to the Amazon page for the book that you wish to review.

Thank you for reading.

~ Ethan Owen

About The Author

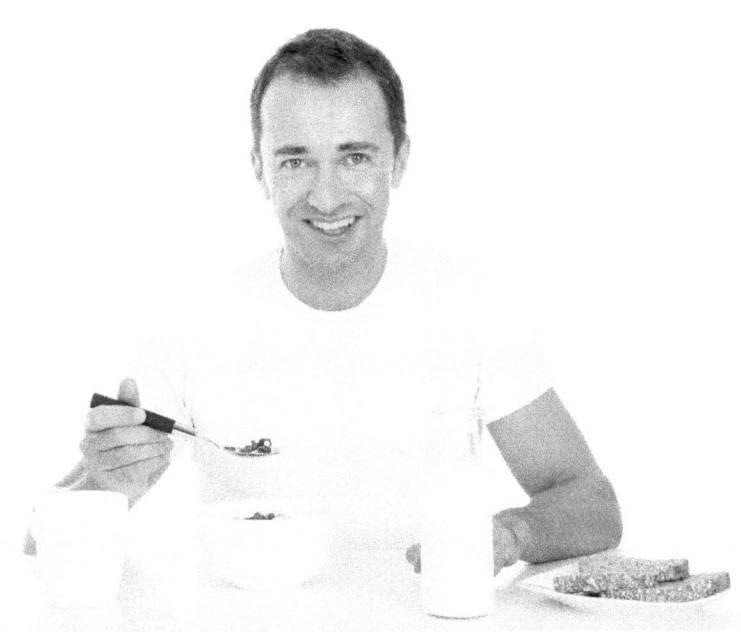

Ethan Owen is a physiotherapist who has always been the healthy eater. This is something that he got from his mother as she always prepared the healthiest meals that she could for her family. However, he never listens to his mother until much later.

Earlier on, Ethan had been bothered by his obesity for years. He struggled with his cravings and could not find a way to effectively get his weight down. The problem was that the more he exercised, the more he guzzled down the calories. It was not until he decided to be a healthy eater. He follows a specific regime to curb his calorie intake and bust his sugar cravings that he was able to start losing the pounds. Ethan documented his success of being able to bust his sugar cravings and you can now follow along with his exact steps to end your addiction in just a few days.

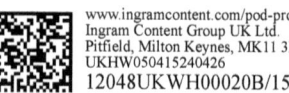
www.ingramcontent.com/pod-product-compliance
Ingram Content Group UK Ltd.
Pitfield, Milton Keynes, MK11 3LW, UK
UKHW050415240426
12048UKWH00020B/1519